Trends in Disease: Volume 1, Issue 1

Prostate Cancer: 2009

Capturing the current trend in prostate cancer therapy and its demographics using lexical statistics

by Kosi Gramatikoff, PhD
Department of Statistics
Burnham Institute for Medical Research
La Jolla, California

Content

I0484966

Conclusions

Generic search with 'prostate cancer' (PC) using semantic utilities such as GoPubMed cannot not reveal automatically to the naive reader what is the current trend in PC therapy. Lexically driven extractions combined with hierarchical clustering point out the focus and current trend - **brachytherapy.**[1] The year 2009 shows an increase of European research on prostate cancer (Table 1).

(1) Koukourakis G *et al.*, Brachytherapy for Prostate Cancer: A Systematic Review of Clinical and Cost Effectiveness, European Urology 2009: 44(1) pp.40-51.

MOTIVATION: Male cancer prevalent cases (5-years: 11,547,465)

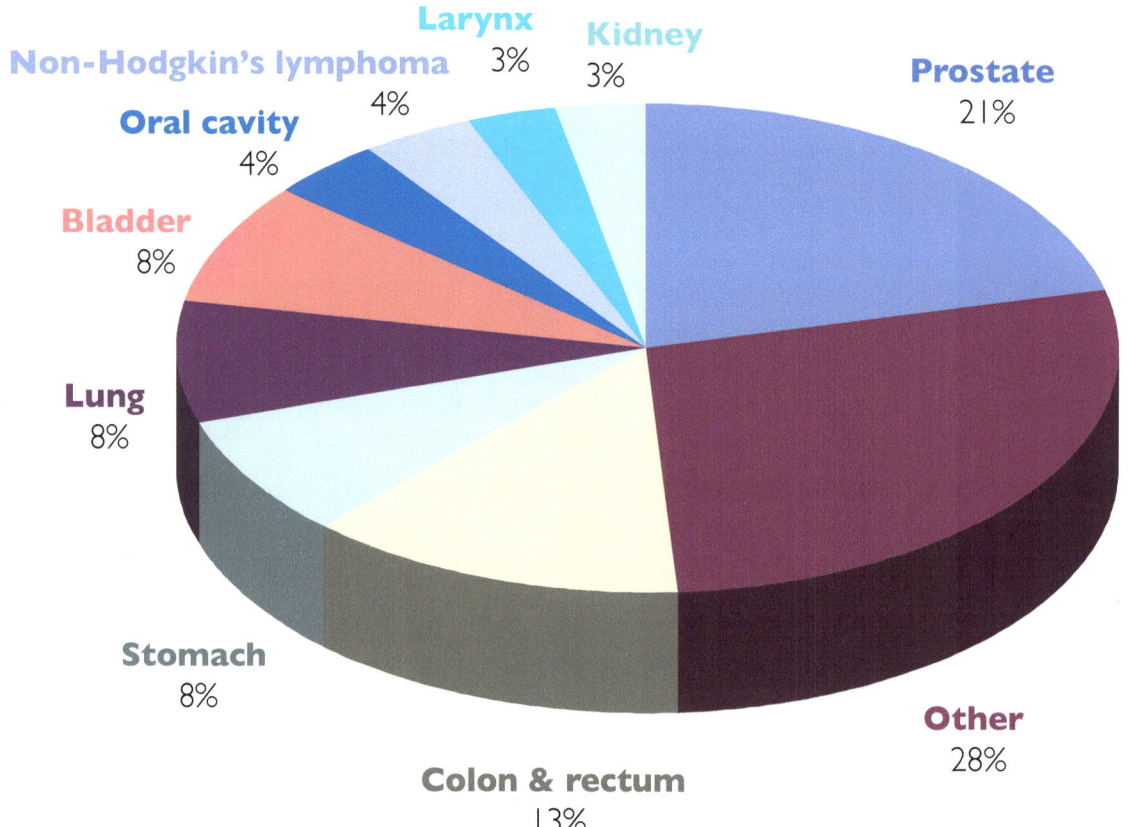

Distribution (%) of cancer types among males diagnosed in last 5 years, global estimate 2002 [Ferlay et al., eds. Globocan 2002: Cancer Incidence, Mortality and Prevalence Worldwide. Lyon France: IARC Press, 2004]

Source of 'prostate cancer' publications: PubMed

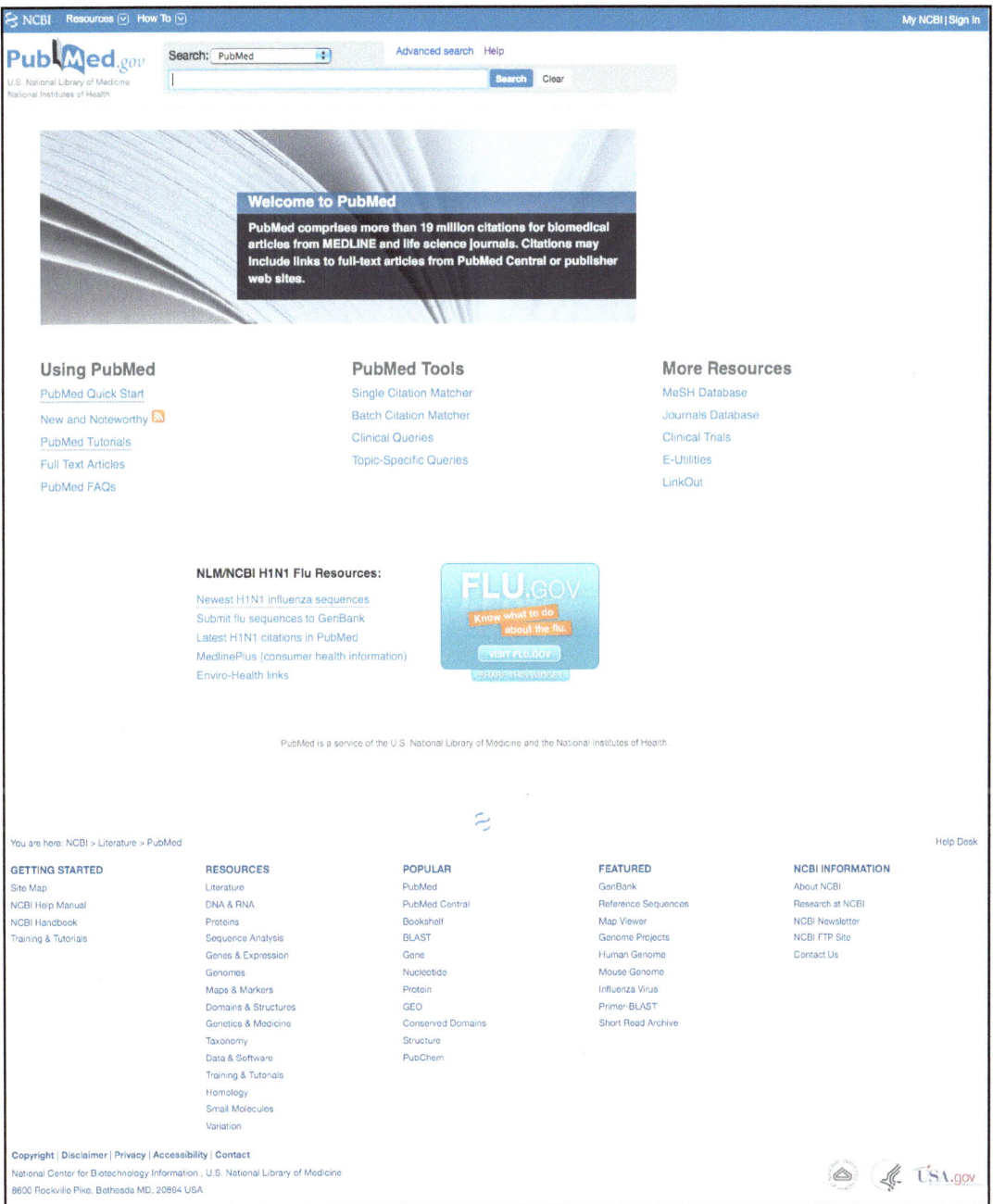

http://www.ncbi.nlm.nih.gov

Search for 'prostate cancer' publications - total: 83,663

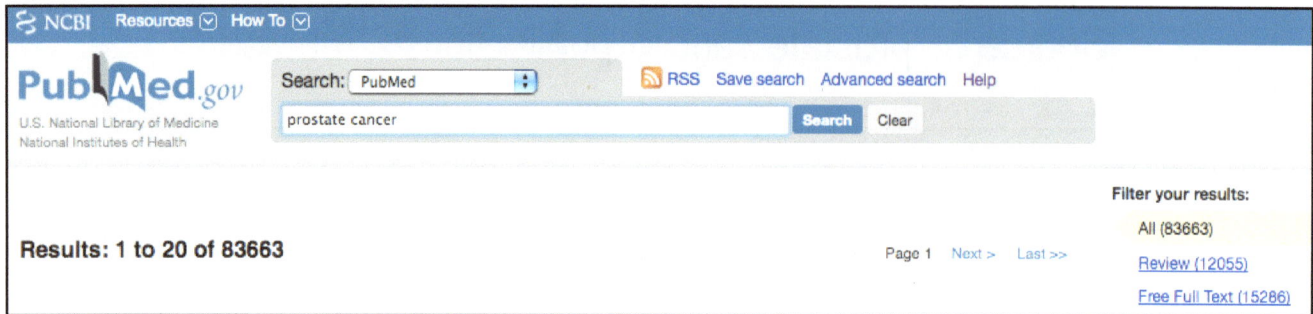

Search for 'prostate cancer' publications in title and abstract - total: 5,715

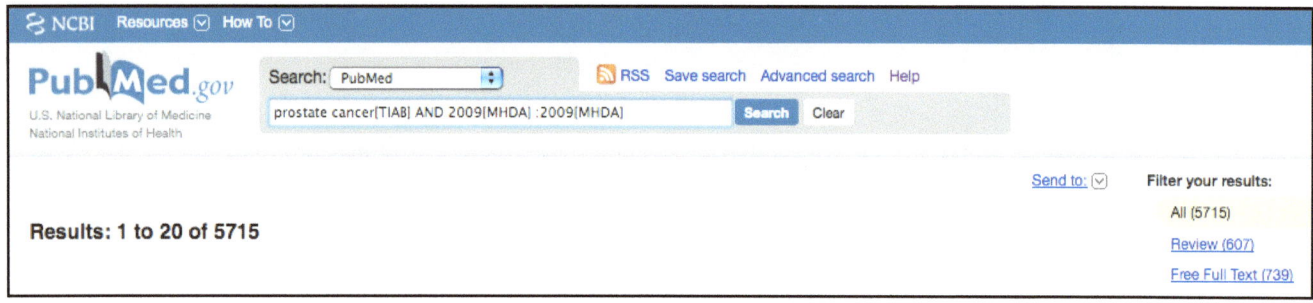

Search for 'prostate cancer' publications in title only - total: 3,704

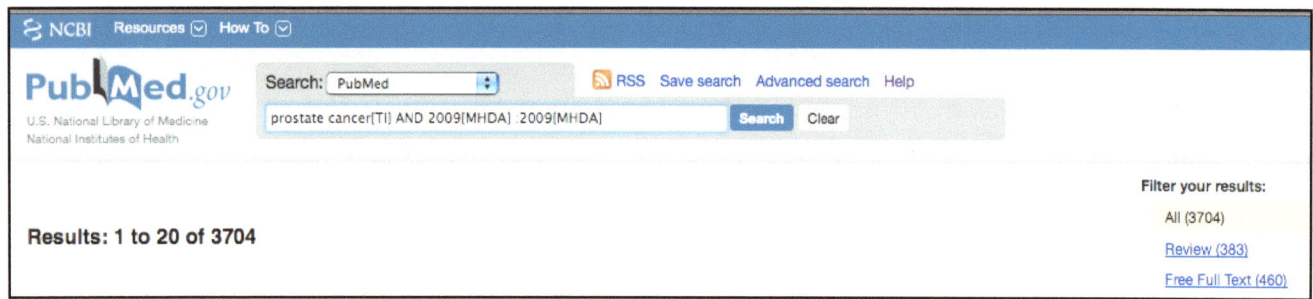

http://www.ncbi.nlm.nih.gov

Top 2,000 PMIDs (2009) were used in phase-I of this study (see Appendix A)

'Prostate cancer' publications over time

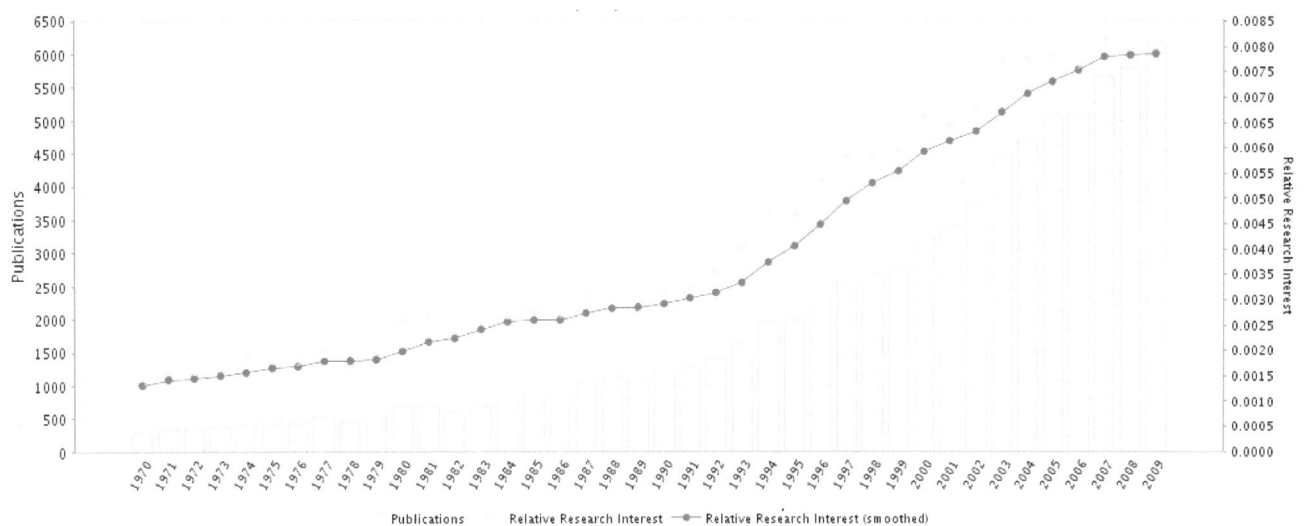

'Prostate cancer' publications on the world map

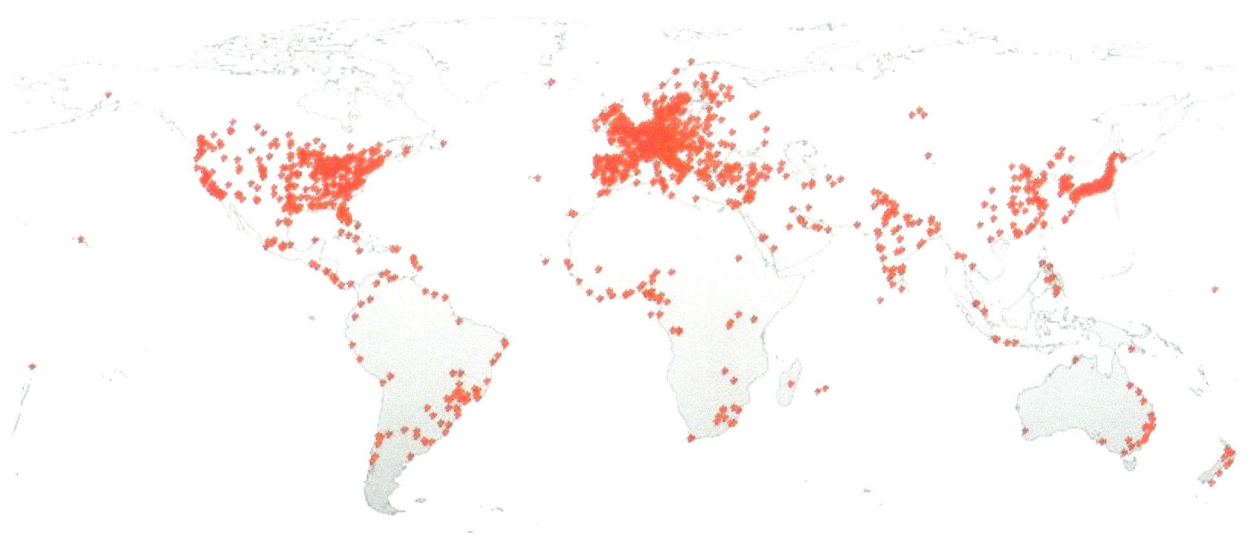

83,663 publications semantically analyzed (www.gopubmed.com)

'Prostate cancer' publications through 40 years (1969-2009)

Top Years	Publications	
2009		6,211
2008		5,794
2007		5,672
2006		5,091
2005		5,058
2004		4,733
2003		4,454
2002		3,733
2001		3,394
2000		3,289
1999		2,784
1998		2,662
1997		2,584
1996		2,282
1995		1,979
1994		1,966
1993		1,634
1992		1,405
1991		1,268
1990		1,213
1988		1,120
1987		1,065
1989		1,060
1985		890
1986		881
1984		775
1983		695
1980		694
1981		665
1982		594
1979		528
1977		519
1978		451
1976		427
1975		427
1974		423
1973		372
1972		337
1971		337
1969		319

83,663 publications semantically analyzed (www.gopubmed.com)

'Prostate cancer' publications by the ttop 40 countries (1909-2009)

Top Countries	Publications	
USA		29,895
Japan		4,365
United Kingdom		3,411
Germany		3,273
Canada		2,721
Italy		2,348
France		2,195
Netherlands		1,553
China		1,401
Sweden		1,364
Spain		1,276
Australia		995
Finland		624
Belgium		606
Austria		572
Switzerland		520
South Korea		449
Taiwan		428
Israel		404
Greece		389
Turkey		389
Norway		377
India		356
Denmark		340
Brazil		330
Ireland		183
Poland		179
New Zealand		137
Czech Republic		136
Hungary		98
Singapore		94
Mexico		84
Portugal		84
South Africa		73
Croatia		70
Russia		67
Iran		65
Hong Kong S.A.R.,		64
Venezuela		61
Argentina		53

Prostate cancer publicationsin in the top 40 journals (1909-2009)

Top Journals	Publications
J Urology	4,430
Urology	3,279
Prostate	2,595
Cancer Res	2,176
Cancer	1,837
Eur Urol	1,767
Int J Radiat Oncol	1,668
Bju Int	1,491
Clin Cancer Res	911
Int J Cancer	893
Br J Urol	833
Hinyokika Kiyo	797
Anticancer Res	675
J Clin Oncol	628
Nippon Hinyokika Gakkai	592
Urologe A	581
Brit J Cancer	545
Urol Int	534
Actas Urol Esp	529
Oncogene	528
J Natl Cancer I	494
Int J Urol	492
Cancer Epidem Biomar	486
Prog Clin Biol Res	477
Radiother Oncol	452
J Biol Chem	450
Arch Esp Urol	432
J Urol	398
Prog Urol	388
Med Phys	340
Cancer Lett	331
Urol Clin N Am	326
Eur J Cancer	320
J Steroid Biochem	314
Jama-j Am Med Assoc	311
Scand J Urol Nephrol	309
Prostate Cancer P D	302
Urol Oncol-semin Ori	300
Nippon Rinsho	300
Int Urol Nephrol	297

83,663 publications semantically analyzed (www.gopubmed.com)

Top 40 generic terms in prostate cancer publicationsin (1909-2009)

Top Terms	Publications
M Prostatic Neoplasms	76,724
M Humans	74,282
M Prostate	73,627
M Prostatitis	73,214
M Prostatism	73,163
M Patients	34,895
M Aged	28,166
M Neoplasms	26,567
M Middle Aged	26,242
M Carcinoma	17,648
M Prostate-Specific Antigen	16,989
M Evaluation Studies as Topic	15,335
M Antigens	14,626
M Men	12,477
M Prostatectomy	12,292
M Adenocarcinoma	12,280
M Diagnosis	12,145
M Neoplasm Metastasis	11,587
M Tissues	11,386
M Animals	11,311
M Adult	10,788
M Proteins	9,668
M Androgens	9,190
M Biopsy	9,116
M Genes	9,017
M Hormones	9,012
M Aged, 80 and over	8,853
P psa	8,773
M Serum	8,314
M Cell Line	8,041
M Neoplasm Staging	7,575
M Breast Neoplasms	7,391
M Prostatic Hyperplasia	7,034
M Prognosis	6,823
M Incidence	6,308
M Radiation	5,977
M Mice	5,908
M Tumor Cells, Cultured	5,774
M Radiotherapy	5,773
M Therapeutics	5,764

83,663 publications semantically analyzed (www.gopubmed.com)

Top 100 terms in 'prostate cancer' publications in (2009: 2,000PMIDs)

Rank	Frequency	Words	Rank	Frequency	Words
1	7613	prostate	55	448	receptor treated
2	7296	cancer	56	447	time
3	3272	patients	57	425	level
4	2315	cells	58	419	respectively
5	1493	men	59	418	cancers
6	1418	expression	60	416	< prostate-specific
7	1397	treatment	61	412	months
8	1393	cell	62	406	association bone
10	1238	study	63	403	serum
11	1197	risk	64	401	high
12	1128	psa	65	400	age radiotherapy
13	962	tumor	66	393	among
14	885	using	67	391	use
15	880	therapy	68	386	genes tissue
16	825	results:	69	385	apoptosis found tumors
18	814	associated	70	383	patient potential
19	767	clinical	71	382	during
20	766	disease	73	373	score
21	761	levels	75	368	factors
22	718	analysis	76	366	screening
23	704	growth	77	361	lncap
24	684	increased	78	357	biochemical
25	677	significantly	79	350	radiation
27	668	human	80	343	stage
28	661	methods:	81	340	toxicity
29	645	compared	82	337	proliferation
30	643	androgen significant	83	335	median
31	634	antigen	84	334	metastatic
32	623	survival	85	332	model
33	622	used	86	330	positive prostatic
34	612	gene	87	329	target
35	609	data	88	327	diagnosis identified
36	599	studies	89	322	volume
37	598	prostatectomy	90	321	development
38	576	activity	91	320	normal
39	569	radical	92	319	rate
40	562	pca	93	314	observed
41	559	biopsy	94	312	localized total
42	537	conclusions: years	95	310	breast low
44	512	progression	96	307	detection
45	509	protein	97	306	background:
46	489	higher	98	305	conclusion: function
47	479	group	99	303	recurrence
48	477	dose	100	301	purpose:
50	461	specific	101	299	further
51	460	gleason	102	296	response
52	459	showed	103	295	findings
53	452	effect	104	292	including
54	449	effects role	105	290	evaluated follow-up increase lower

Total words analyzed: 3,055,346

Ten-(10)-term signature tested for 'prostate cancer' researchers (2009: 2,000PMIDs)

Rank	Frequency	Terms
15	880	therapy
37	598	prostatectomy
65	400	radiotherapy
84	334	metastatic
88	327	diagnosis
148	212	brachytherapy
156	202	surgical
187	165	carcinoma
216	134	docetaxel
217	133	chemotherapy

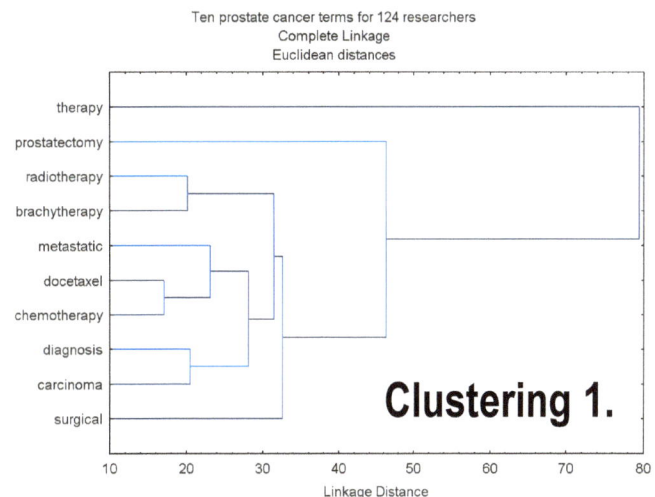

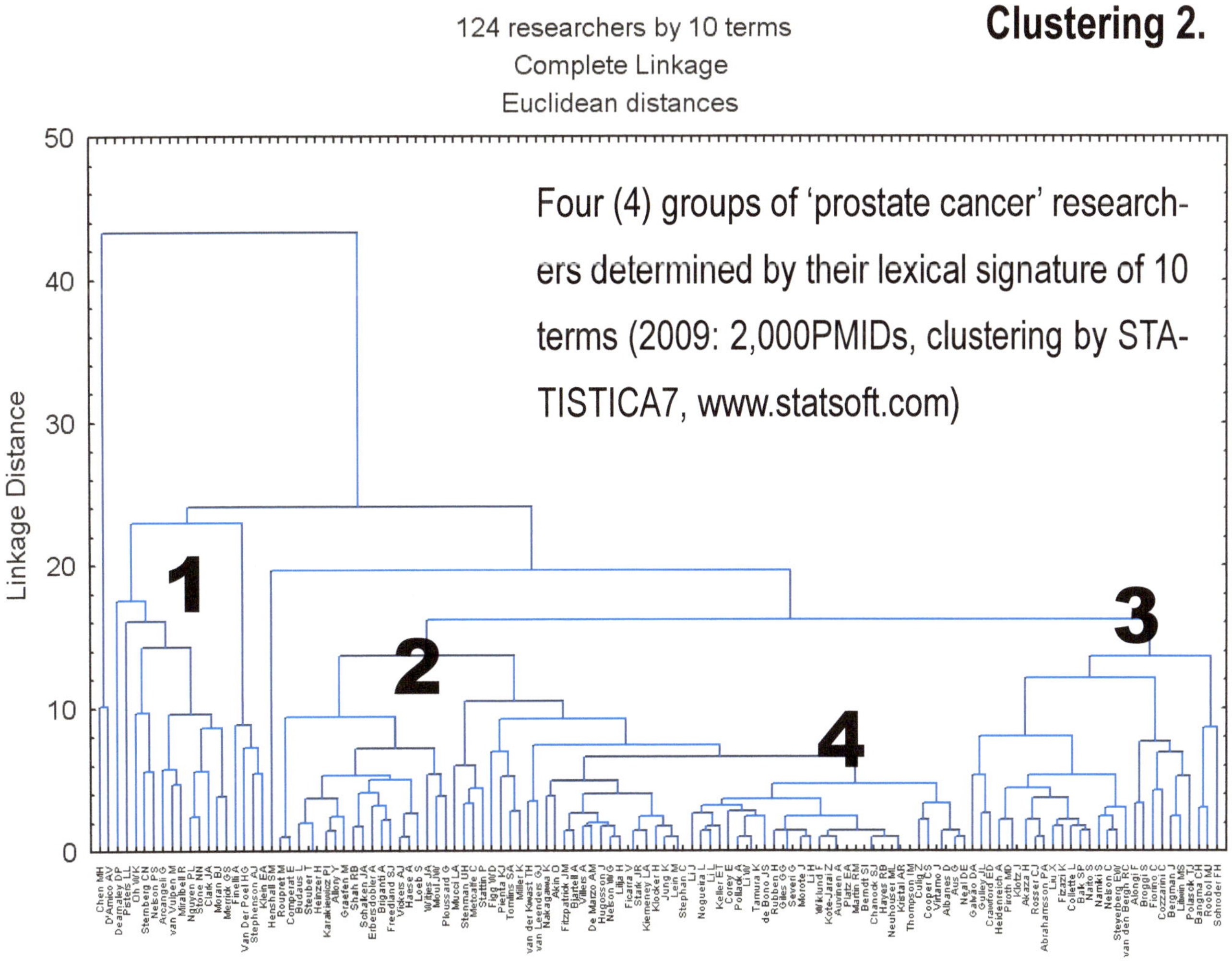

Ten prostate cancer terms for 124 researchers
Complete Linkage
Euclidean distances
therapy
prostatectomy
radiotherapy
brachytherapy
metastatic
docetaxel
chemotherapy
diagnosis
carcinoma
surgical
Clustering 1.
10 20 30 40 50 60 70 80
Linkage Distance

124 researchers by 10 terms
Complete Linkage
Euclidean distances
Clustering 2.
Linkage Distance
0 10 20 30 40 50
1
2
3
4
Four (4) groups of 'prostate cancer' researchers determined by their lexical signature of 10 terms (2009: 2,000PMIDs, clustering by STATISTICA7, www.statsoft.com)

Rank and counts of researchers (2009: 2000PMIDs, page 1)

E-rank	Total PubMed	therapy	prosta-tectomy	radio-therapy	meta-static	diagnosis	brachy-therapy	surgical	carci-noma	docetaxel	chemo-therapy	total Whits	Name
18	300	9	4	1	7	8	0	2	4	0	0	35	Schroder FH
14	181	39	4	6	0	3	14	4	2	0	0	72	D'Amico AV
13	73	4	3	1	0	8	0	2	4	0	0	22	Roobol MJ
11	63	32	1	5	0	2	9	0	1	0	0	50	Chen MH
11	78	6	5	2	0	8	0	2	4	0	0	27	Bangma CH
10	98	0	1	0	0	2	0	0	0	0	0	3	Neal DE
10	11	4	10	0	0	1	0	4	1	0	0	20	Ploussard G
10	60	1	3	0	5	0	0	0	2	0	0	11	Miller K
10	65	3	8	0	1	1	0	3	0	0	0	16	Loeb S
9	76	0	0	0	0	3	0	0	0	0	0	3	Albanes D
9	153	7	8	2	3	2	3	12	0	0	0	37	Klein EA
9	59	11	7	1	1	0	4	3	0	0	0	27	Polascik TJ
9	206	0	0	0	0	0	0	1	0	0	0	1	Thompson IM
8	218	6	7	0	1	1	0	3	1	0	0	19	Moul JW
8	113	0	0	0	3	5	0	1	0	0	0	9	Stattin P
8	18	5	3	1	0	2	0	2	0	0	0	13	van den Bergh RC
8	102	2	8	1	0	1	0	1	0	0	0	13	Freedland SJ
7	95	1	3	0	0	0	0	0	2	0	0	6	Stephan C
7	20	0	0	0	0	0	0	0	0	0	0	8	Metcalfe C
7	19	9	10	4	1	0	0	0	0	0	0	24	Cozzarini C
7	29	10	6	5	1	0	0	0	0	0	0	22	Fiorino C
7	34	3	3	0	1	4	0	2	4	0	0	17	van Leenders GJ
7	82	14	1	1	0	1	9	0	1	0	0	27	Merrick GS
7	141	4	6	0	0	2	0	2	0	0	0	14	Graefen M
7	70	0	0	0	0	0	0	0	0	0	0	0	Hayes RB
7	129	11	6	4	0	0	5	0	0	0	0	26	Litwin MS
7	28	0	0	0	0	1	0	0	0	0	0	1	Martin RM
6	49	0	0	0	0	0	0	1	0	0	0	1	Kristal AR
6	24	0	0	0	0	0	0	0	0	0	0	0	Chanock SJ
6	25	2	0	2	1	3	0	0	0	0	0	8	Cooper CS
6	13	5	2	1	0	2	0	0	0	0	0	10	Steyerberg EW
6	12	1	7	0	0	0	0	5	7	0	0	20	Comperat E
6	102	0	0	0	0	1	0	0	0	0	0	1	Platz EA
6	80	1	8	0	0	0	0	2	0	0	0	11	Haese A
6	139	0	2	0	0	1	0	0	0	0	0	3	Lilja H
6	81	1	5	0	1	2	0	0	1	0	0	10	Schalken JA
6	26	2	0	0	1	0	0	0	0	0	2	5	de Bono JS
6	132	1	3	0	0	0	0	0	1	0	0	5	Jung K
6	21	0	5	0	0	6	0	0	0	0	0	11	Mucci LA
6	86	1	3	0	0	0	0	0	2	0	0	6	Lein M
6	53	4	0	0	1	0	0	0	1	0	0	6	Naito S
6	77	11	0	0	3	0	0	0	0	0	6	6	26	Nelson PS
6	29	11	1	4	3	2	2	0	0	0	0	23	Miralbell R
6	49	4	1	0	1	0	0	0	0	0	0	6	Balk SP
6	89	1	0	1	0	5	0	0	0	0	0	7	Stenman UH
6	36	1	8	0	0	0	0	3	0	0	0	12	Vickers AJ
6	147	2	0	0	4	0	0	1	0	5	0	12	Figg WD
6	20	4	5	0	0	1	0	1	1	0	0	12	Allory Y
5	19	0	0	0	0	0	0	0	0	0	0	0	Berndt SI
5	66	3	7	0	0	0	0	0	0	0	0	10	Briganti A

Rank and counts of researchers (2009: 2000PMIDs, page 2)

E-rank	Total PubMed	therapy	prosta-tectomy	radiothe-rapy	meta-static	diagno-sis	brachy-therapy	surgical	carcino-ma	doceta-xel	chemo-therapy	total Whits	Name
5	232	6	0	0	5	0	0	0	1	0	0	12	Crawford ED
5	107	10	0	5	11	0	0	0	0	0	0	26	Dearnaley DP
5	44	2	0	0	1	0	0	0	0	2	0	5	Corey E
5	51	3	8	0	2	1	0	1	2	1	3	21	Witjes JA
5	50	8	0	0	6	0	0	0	0	1	0	15	Gulley JL
5	70	0	0	0	0	2	0	0	0	0	0	2	Aus G
5	26	7	6	3	0	1	0	7	0	0	0	24	Van Der Poel HG
5	43	0	0	0	0	3	0	0	0	0	0	3	Virtamo J
5	8	6	0	2	0	0	3	0	0	0	0	11	Klotz J
5	72	18	10	1	0	2	0	1	0	0	1	33	Pisters LL
5	21	6	0	2	0	0	3	0	0	0	0	11	Piroth MD
5	34	1	6	0	0	0	0	5	7	0	0	19	Roupret M
5	141	4	5	0	0	1	0	0	0	0	0	10	Karakiewicz PI
5	34	4	10	2	0	0	1	12	0	0	0	29	Stephenson AJ
5	79	17	0	0	1	2	0	0	0	2	9	31	Oh WK
5	83	2	0	0	1	2	0	0	0	0	0	5	Culig Z
4	71	2	2	0	0	1	0	0	0	0	0	5	De Marzo AM
4	11	0	3	0	0	0	0	4	0	0	0	7	Akin O
4	43	1	3	0	1	1	0	1	0	0	0	7	Bjartell A
4	48	0	0	0	0	1	0	0	0	0	0	1	Auvinen A
4	15	14	2	4	0	0	0	0	0	0	0	20	Arcangeli G
4	44	0	3	0	0	0	0	1	0	0	0	4	Kiemeney LA
4	10	16	0	3	0	0	7	0	0	0	0	26	Moran BJ
4	9	7	3	2	0	0	0	0	0	0	0	12	Broggi S
4	32	9	0	0	6	1	0	0	0	2	7	25	Sternberg CN
4	105	0	0	0	1	0	0	0	1	0	0	2	Li H
4	63	1	0	0	2	0	0	0	0	0	0	3	Keller ET
4	7	7	6	3	1	0	0	0	0	0	0	17	Alongi F
4	29	3	0	1	0	0	0	0	0	0	0	4	Fizazi K
4	62	0	0	0	0	1	0	1	0	0	0	2	Wiklund F
4	41	0	0	0	0	1	0	0	1	0	0	2	Severi G
4	73	1	0	0	2	0	0	0	2	0	0	5	Li J
4	49	0	0	0	0	1	0	0	1	0	0	2	Giles GG
4	22	3	5	0	0	0	0	2	0	0	0	10	Heinzer H
4	98	0	4	0	0	0	0	0	2	0	0	6	Klocker H
4	28	0	0	0	0	0	0	0	2	0	0	2	Rubben H
4	10	1	0	0	0	0	0	0	0	0	0	1	Tamura K
4	29	8	1	1	0	2	6	0	0	0	0	18	Clark JA
4	7	9	5	4	0	0	4	0	0	0	0	22	Bergman J
4	51	0	0	0	0	0	0	0	1	0	0	1	Morote J
4	79	1	1	1	0	1	0	0	0	0	0	4	Hugosson J
4	201	0	0	0	6	0	0	0	0	0	0	6	Pienta KJ
4	10	1	5	0	0	0	0	2	0	0	0	8	Budaus L
4	42	5	0	1	1	0	0	0	0	0	0	7	Collette L
4	91	0	1	0	1	0	0	0	0	0	0	2	Li L
4	96	4	0	0	0	0	0	0	0	0	1	5	Liu X
4	37	1	0	0	0	0	0	0	0	0	0	1	Li W
4	22	11	0	6	0	0	4	0	0	0	0	21	van Vulpen M
4	18	0	0	0	0	0	0	1	0	0	0	1	Neuhouser ML
4	21	1	2	0	0	0	0	2	0	3	0	8	Nakagawa K

Rank and counts of researchers (2009: 2000PMIDs, page 3)

E-rank	Total PubMed	therapy	prosta-tectomy	radiothe-rapy	meta-static	diagno-sis	brachy-therapy	surgical	carcino-ma	doceta-xel	chemo-therapy	total Whits	Name
4	36	5	2	1	0	0	0	0	0	0	0	8	Namiki S
4	63	5	1	0	0	2	0	0	0	0	0	8	Nelson C
4	90	12	0	2	0	0	3	0	0	0	0	17	Stone NN
4	4	1	1	0	1	0	0	1	0	0	0	4	Nogueira L
4	61	5	0	0	0	0	0	0	0	0	0	5	Abrahamsson PA
4	20	11	0	1	0	0	5	0	0	0	0	17	Nguyen PL
4	60	1	2	0	1	1	0	0	2	0	0	7	Fitzpatrick JM
4	43	1	6	0	2	2	0	0	2	0	0	13	Shah RB
4	30	2	1	0	3	0	0	0	1	15	2	24	Henshall SM
4	9	0	4	0	0	0	0	0	0	0	0	4	Stark JR
4	40	3	5	0	0	0	0	2	0	0	0	10	Steuber T
4	100	0	2	0	4	0	3	4	0	0	0	13	van der Kwast TH
4	32	0	4	0	3	1	0	0	1	0	0	9	Tomlins SA
4	17	0	4	0	0	0	0	0	0	0	0	4	Ficarra V
4	19	0	0	0	0	1	0	0	0	0	0	1	Kote-Jarai Z
3	11	7	11	7	0	0	0	13	0	0	0	38	Finelli A
3	171	2	0	0	0	0	0	0	0	0	0	2	Pollack A
3	112	6	0	0	2	0	0	0	0	0	0	8	Akaza H
3	63	0	8	0	0	0	0	0	0	0	0	8	Erbersdobler A
3	68	1	3	1	0	1	0	0	0	0	0	6	Villers A
3	37	5	0	0	0	0	3	0	0	0	0	8	Heidenreich A
3	76	1	2	0	0	1	0	0	0	0	0	4	Nelson WG
3	43	6	0	0	0	0	0	0	0	0	0	6	Rosser CJ
3	10	9	0	0	1	1	0	0	0	0	0	11	Galvão DA

'Brachytherapy' term is emerging from comparison of 19 researchers' 1,026 publications from **Clustering 2** (cluster#1, left).

Arcangeli G
Chen MH
Clark JA
D'Amico AV
Dearnaley DP
Finelli A
Klein EA
Merrick GS
Miralbell R
Moran BJ
Nelson PS
Nguyen PL
Oh WK
Pisters LL
Stephenson AJ
Sternberg CN
Stone NN
Van Der Poel HG
van Vulpen M

Rank1	Frequency1	Rank2	Frequency2	Terms	F-increase
148	212	28	562	brachytherapy	2.651
217	133	111	191	chemotherapy	1.436
65	400	29	554	radiotherapy	1.385
15	880	8	1094	therapy	1.243
37	598	17	636	prostatectomy	1.064
216	134	158	130	docetaxel	0.970
156	202	116	185	surgical	0.916
187	165	172	110	carcinoma	0.667
84	334	101	208	metastatic	0.623
88	327	124	172	diagnosis	0.526

1,026 PMIDs analyzed (extracted by the 19 names, left)

Top 40 terms/authors 'brachytherapy AND prostate cancer' (1909-2009)

Top Terms	Publications		Top Authors	Publications	
M Brachytherapy	2,795		Wallner K	153	
M Prostatic Neoplasms	2,768		Merrick G	135	
M Humans	2,676		Butler W	134	
M Prostate	2,663		Stock R	74	
M Prostatism	2,659		Stone N	68	
M Prostatitis	2,659		Galbreath R	61	
M Patients	1,977		Lief J	52	
M Aged	1,055		Martinez A	48	
M Radiation	1,023		Blasko J	44	
M Middle Aged	923		Zelefsky M	36	
M Radiotherapy	792		Potters L	35	
M Radiotherapy Dosage	761		Roach M	34	
M Prostate-Specific Antigen	748		Grimm P	33	
M Iodine Radioisotopes	736		Allen Z	31	
M Evaluation Studies as Topic	730		Adamovich E	30	
M Prostatectomy	647		Cavanagh W	30	
M Antigens	554		Pouliot J	28	
M Treatment Outcome	492		Sutlief S	28	
M Neoplasms	469		D'Amico A	27	
M Follow-Up Studies	440		Zaider M	26	
M Neoplasm Staging	433		Schellhammer P	26	
M Men	430		Crook J	25	
M Adenocarcinoma	427		Davis B	24	
M Carcinoma	411		Waterman F	24	
M Hormones	388		Vicini F	24	
M Methods	374		Langley S	23	
M Aged, 80 and over	372		Gustafson G	23	
M Biopsy	362		Edmundson G	23	
M Morbidity	350		Kattan M	22	
P psa	336		Theodorescu D	22	
M Radioisotopes	304		Laing R	21	
M Recurrence	300		Tempany C	21	
M Combined Modality Therapy	296		Dorsey A	21	
M Radiotherapy Planning, Compι	294		Carroll P	20	
M Disease-Free Survival	282		Dicker A	20	
M Therapeutics	276		Kuban D	20	
M Palladium	272		Sylvester J	20	
M Needles	270		Beyer D	20	
M Tomography, X-Ray Computec	266		Ciezki J	19	
M Androgens	264		Battermann J	19	

2,821 publications semantically analyzed (www.gopubmed.com)

'Brachytherapy AND prostate cancer' publications over time

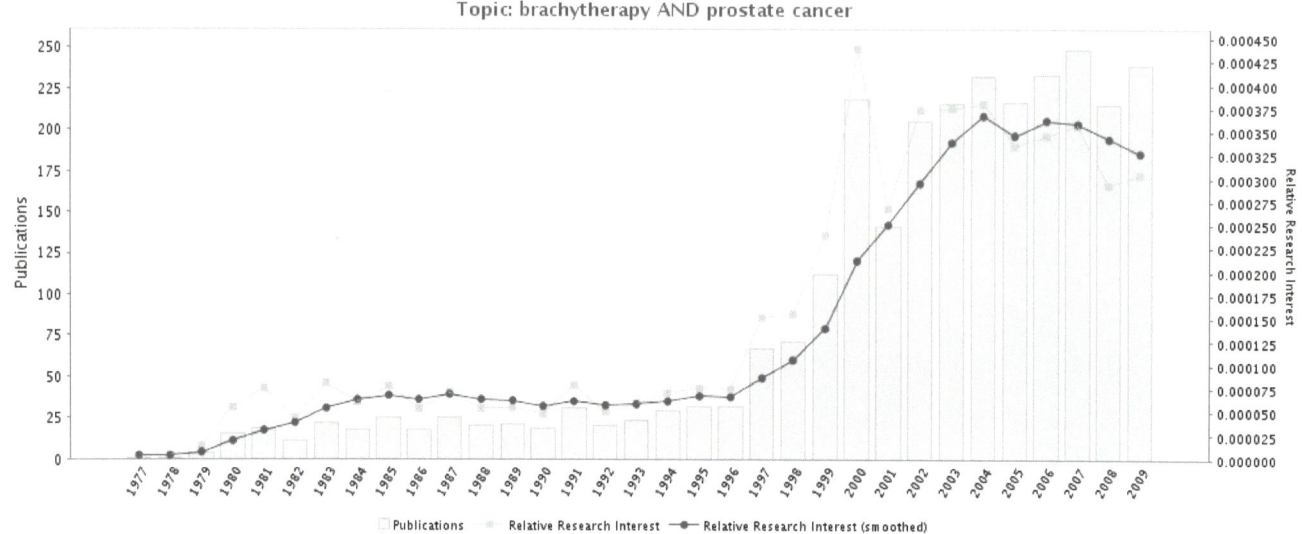

Topic: brachytherapy AND prostate cancer

'Brachytherapy AND prostate cancer' publications on the world map

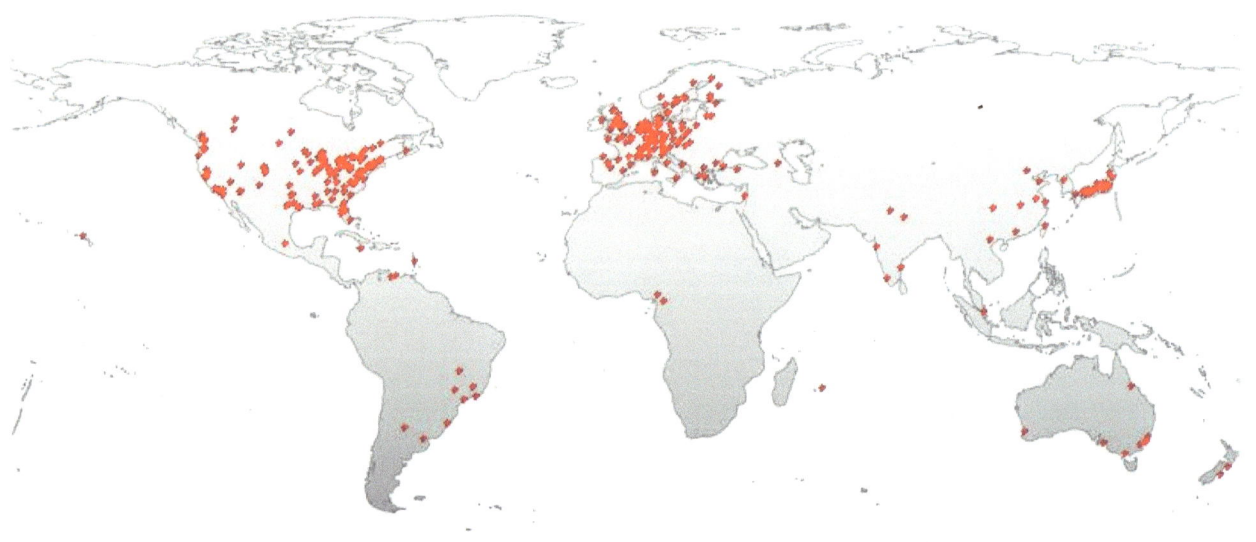

2,821 publications semantically analyzed (www.gopubmed.com)

Authors network on 'brachytherapy AND prostate cancer' (1909-2009). Yellow nodes are authors matching the initial set (Appendix A.) and show higher activity in year 2009 (

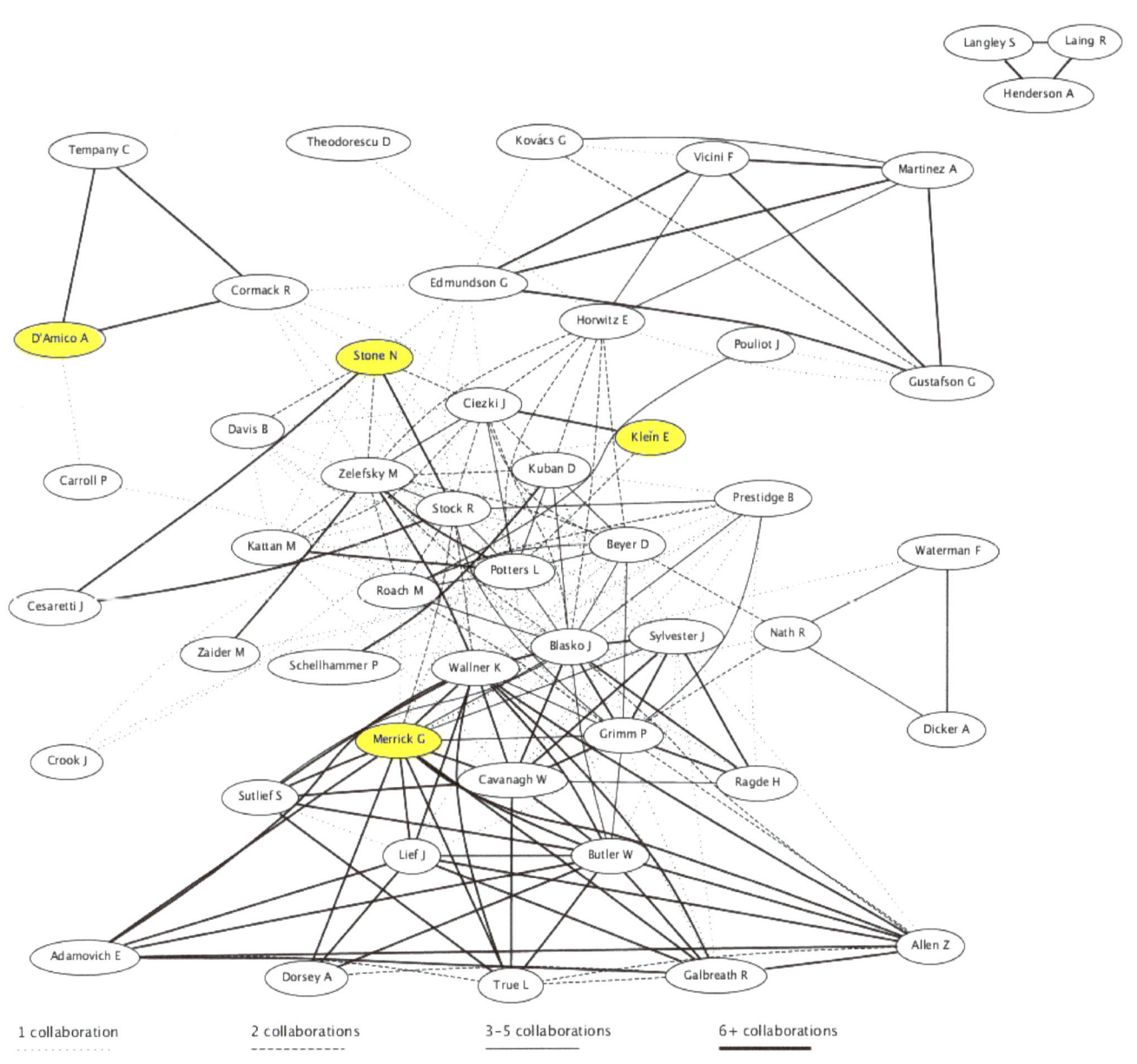

1 collaboration · · · · · · · · ·   2 collaborations - - - - - - -   3–5 collaborations ———   6+ collaborations ▬▬▬

2,821 publications semantically analyzed (www.gopubmed.com)

List 1. Alphabetical list of top ranked participants for year 2009 (page 1)

Name	Email	Institution
Abrahamsson PA	Per-Anders.Abrahamsson@skane.se	Malmö University Hospital, Malmö, Sweden.
Akaza H	akazah@md.tsukuba.ac.jp	Sapporo Medical University School of Medicine dDepartment of Urology
Akin O	akino@mskcc.org	Department of Radiology, Memorial Sloan-Kettering Cancer Center, 1275 York Avenue, room C-278, New York, NY, 10065, USA.
Albanes D	daa@nih.gov	Nutritional Epidemiology Branch, Division of Cancer Epidemiology and Genetics, National Cancer Institute, 6120 Executive Blvd, Rm 3044, Bethesda, MD 20892-7242, USA
Allory Y	yves.allory@hmn.aphp.fr	INSERM U955 Eq07 Department of Urology, APHP, CHU Henri Mondor, Créteil, France
Alongi F	filippo.alongi@hsr.it	Department of Radiotherapy, Scientific Institute H San Raffaele, Milan, Italy.
Arcangeli G	arcangeli@ifo.it	Department of Radiotherapy, Regina Elena National Cancer Institute, Rome, Italy
Aus G	gunnar.aus@vgregion.se	Department of Urology, Sahlgrenska University Hospital, Gothenburg, Sweden.
Auvinen A	ansii.auvinen@utu.fi	School of Public Health, University of Tampere, FIN-33014 Tampere, Finland
Balk SP	sbalk@caregroup.harvard.edu	Beth Israel Deaconess Medical Center, 330 Brookline Avenue, Boston, MA 02115
Bangma CH	h.j.vanalphen@erasmusmc.nl	Department of Urology, Erasmus Medical Center, Rotterdam, The Netherlands, www.eur.nl/english/
Bergman J	jbergman@mednet.ucla.edu	Department of Urology, University of California at Los Angeles, Los Angeles, California 90095-1738, USA
Berndt SI	berndts@mail.nih.gov	Laboratory of Translational Genomics, Division of Cancer Epidemiology and Genetics, National Cancer Institute, National Institutes of Health, 8717 Grovemont Circle, Gaithersburg, MD, 20877
Bjartell A	anders.bjartell@kir.mas.lu.se	Department of Clinical Sciences, Division of Urological Cancers, Clinical Research Center, University Hospital Malmö, Lund University, Malmö, Sweden.
Briganti A	briganti_alberto@yahoo.it	Department of Urology, Vita-Salute University, San Raffaele Hospital, Via Olgettina, 60, 20132, Milan, Italy.
Broggi S	broggi.sara@hsr.it	Department of Medical Physics, San Raffaele Scientific Institute, Milan, Italy
Budaus L	Lars_budaeus@web.de	Martini-Clinic, Prostate Cancer Centre Hamburg-Eppendorf, Hamburg, Germany
Chanock SJ	chanocks@mail.nih.gov	Laboratory of Translational Genomics, Division of Cancer Epidemiology and Genetics, National Cancer Institute, National Institutes of Health, Department of Health and Human Services, Bethesda, Maryland
Chen MH	rcchen@partners.org	Harvard Radiation Oncology Program, Harvard Medical School, Boston, MA, USA
Clark JA	jaclark@bu.edu	Center for Health Quality, Outcomes, and Economic Research, Edith Nourse Rogers Memorial Veterans Hospital, Bedford, US

List 1. Alphabetical list of top ranked participants for year 2009 (page 2)

Name	Email	Institution
Collette L	laurence.collette@eortc.be	Statistics Department, European Organisation for Research and Treatment of Cancer Data Center, Brussels, Belgium
Comperat E	ecomperat@yahoo.fr	Department of Pathology, Pitie-Salpetriere Hospital, GHU Est, University PMC Paris VI, Paris, France
Cooper CS	colin.cooper@icr.ac.uk	Male Urological Cancer Research Centre, Sutton, UK
Corey E	ecorey@u.washington.edu	Department of Urology, University of Washington, 1959 NE Pacific Street, Seattle, WA 98195, USA.
Cozzarini C	cozzarini.cesare@hsr.it	Department of Radiotherapy, Scientific Institute Hospital San Raffaele, Medical Physics, IRCCS S. Raffaele, Milano, Italy
Crawford ED	david.crawford@uchsc.edu	Section of Urologic Oncology, University of Colorado Health Science Center, Denver, Colorado, USA.
Culig Z	zoran.culig@uibk.ac.at	Department of Urology, Innsbruck Medical University, Anichstrasse 35, A-6020 Innsbruck, Austria.
D'Amico AV	adamico@partners.org	Department of Radiation Oncology, Brigham and Women's Hospital, Boston, MA 02215, USA.
de Bono JS	jdebono@icr.ac.uk	Section of Medicine and Cancer Research UK Centre for Cancer Therapeutics, The Institute of Cancer Research and Royal Marsden NHS Foundation Trust, Sutton, Surrey SM2 5PT, United Kingdom
De Marzo AM	ademarz@jhmi.edu	Department of Pathology, Sidney Kimmel Comprehensive Cancer Center, and Department of Urology, James Buchanan Brady Urological Institute, Johns Hopkins University School of Medicine, Baltimore, MD 21287
Dearnaley DP	david.dearnaley@icr.ac.uk	Royal Marsden Foundation Trust and Institute of Cancer Research, Sutton, Surrey, UK.
Erbersdobler A	andreas.erbersdobler@ charite.de	Institute of Pathology, Charité University Hospital Berlin, Charitéplatz 1, 10117, Berlin, Germany
Ficarra V	vincenzoficarra@hotmail.com	Department of Urology, University of Verona, Ospedale Policlinico G.B. Rossi, Verona, Italy.
Figg WD	wdfigg@helix.gov	Clinical Pharmacology Program, Medical Oncology Branch, Center for Cancer Research, National Cancer Institute, Bethesda, Maryland, MD, 21702
Finelli A	a.finelli@utoronto.ca	Princess Margaret Hospital, Toronto, Ontario, Canada
Fiorino C	fiorino.claudio@hsr.it	Department of Radiotherapy, Scientific Institute Hospital San Raffaele, Medical Physics, IRCCS S. Raffaele, Milano, Italy
Fitzpatrick JM	profsurg@iol.ie	Department of Surgery, Mater Hospital, Dublin, Ireland
Fizazi K	fizazi@igr.fr	Institut Gustave Roussy, University of Paris XI, Villejuif, France, and Charité, Universitätsmedizin Berlin, Berlin, Germany.
Freedland SJ	steve.freedland@duke.edu	Department of Surgery (Urology), Durham VA Medical Center and Duke Prostate Center, Duke University School of Medicine, Durham, NC 27710
Galvão DA	d.galvao@ecu.edu.au	School of Exercise, Biomedical and Health Sciences, Edith Cowan University, Joondalup, Western Australia

Name	Email	Institution
Giles GG	Graham.Giles@cancervic.org.au	Cancer Epidemiology Centre, The Cancer Council Victoria, Melbourne, Australia.
Graefen M	graefen@uke.uni-hamburg.de	Martini-Clinic, Prostate Cancer Center, University Hospital Hamburg-Eppendorf, Hamburg, Germany.
Gulley JL	gulleyj@mail.nih.gov	Laboratory of Tumor Immunology and Biology,Center for Cancer Research, National Cancer Institute, National Institutes of Health, 10 Center Drive, Room 8B09, Bethesda, MD 20892, USA.
Haese A	haese@uke.uni-hamburg.de	Department of Urology, University Hospital Hamburg-Eppendorf, Hamburg.
Hayes RB	hayesr@mail.nih.gov	Laboratory of Translational Genomics, Division of Cancer Epidemiology and Genetics, National Cancer Institute, National Institutes of Health, 8717 Grovemont Circle, Gaithersburg, MD, 20877
Heidenreich A	axel.heidenreich@uk-koeln.de	Bereich Uro-Onkologie,Klinik und Poliklinik für Urologie, Uniklinik, Kerpener Strasse 62, 50924, Köln, Deutschland
Heinzer H	heinzer@uke.uni-hamburg.de	Martini-Klinik, Prostate Cancer Center, University Medical Center Hamburg-Eppendorf, Hamburg, Germany.
Henshall SM	s.henshall@garvan.org.au	Cancer Research Program, Garvan Institute of Medical Research, St Vincent's Hospital, Sydney, NSW 2010, Australia.
Hugosson J	jonas.hugosson@urology.gu.se	Department of Urology, Sahlrenska University Hospital, Gothenburg, Sweden
Jung K	jung@rz.charite.hu-berlin.de	Department of Urology, Charite-Universitätsmedizin Berlin, Berlin, Germany
Karakiewicz PI	pierre.karakiewicz@umontreal.ca	Cancer Prognostics and Health Outcomes Unit, University of Montréal Health Centre (CHUM), Montréal,Montreal, Canada.
Keller ET	etkeller@umich.edu	Department of Urology, University of Michigan Health System, Ann Arbor, Michigan 48109-0654, USA.
Kiemeney LA	b.kiemeney@epib.umcn.nl	Department of Epidemiology and Biostatistics, Radboud University Nijmegen Medical Centre, Nijmegen, the Netherlands.
Klein EA	kleine@ccf.org	Glickman Urological and Kidney Institute, Cleveland Clinic, Cleveland, OH
Klocker H	helmut.klocker@uibk.ac.at	Department of Urology, University of Innsbruck, Austria
Klotz J	judith.klotz@comcast.net	School of Public Health, University of Medicine and Dentistry of New Jersey, Piscataway, NJ, USA.
Kote-Jarai Z	zsofia.kote-jarai@icr.ac.uk	Translational Cancer Genetics Team, The Institute of Cancer Research, Sutton, Surrey, UK
Kristal AR	akristal@fhcrc.org	Fred Hutchinson Cancer Research Center, Cancer Prevention Program, Seattle, Washington.
Lein M	Michael.Lein@charite.de	Department of Urology, Charité Hospital Berlin, Campus Mitte, University Medicine Berlin, Berlin, Germany.
Li H	ctelhh@nccs.com.sg	Biostatistics Unit, Division of Clinical Trials and Epidemiological Sciences, National Cancer Centre, 11 Hospital Drive, Singapore 129610, Singapore.

List 1. Alphabetical list of top ranked participants for year 2009 (page 4)

Name	Email	Institution
Li J	Gongzh@nic.Emi.ac.cn	Institute of Pharmacology and Toxicology, Academy of Military Medical Sciences, Beijing, China.
Li L	li.li@kbh.uu.se	Department of Women's and Children's Health, Division for Obstetrics and Gynecology, Uppsala University, Uppsala, Sweden
Li W	liw1@auhs.edu	Department of Ophthalmology, Allegheny University, Philadelphia, Pa. 19102, USA
Lilja H	Hans.lilja@klkemi.mas.lu.se	Department of Urology, Sahlgrenska University Hospital, Goteborg, Sweden.
Litwin MS	mlitwin@ucla.edu	UCLA Department of Urology, Box 951738, Los Angeles, CA, 90095-1738
Liu X	liu@ch11.ukl.uni-freiburg.de	University Hospital Freiburg, Department of General and Visceral Surgery, University of Freiburg, Freiburg, Germany.
Loeb S	stacyloeb@gmail.com	Brady Urological Institute, Johns Hopkins Medical Institutions, 600 N Wolfe Street, Marburg 1, Baltimore, MD 21287, USA
Martin RM	richard.martin@bristol.ac.uk	Department of Social Medicine, University of Bristol, Bristol, BS8 2PS, UK
Merrick GS	gmerrick@urologicre-searchinstitute.org	Schiffler Cancer Center, Wheeling Jesuit University, Wheeling, WV 26003-6300
Metcalfe C	chris.metcalfe@bristol.ac.uk	Department of Social Medicine, University of Bristol, Canynge Hall, 39 Whatley Road, Bristol, BS8 2PS United Kingdom
Miller K	kurt.miller@charite.de	Department of Urology, Charite-Universitätsmedizin Berlin, Berlin, Germany.
Miralbell R	Raymond.Mirabell@hcuge.ch	Institute for Social and Preventive Medicine, University of Geneva, Geneva, Switzerland.
Moran BJ	brendan.moran@nhht.nhs.uk	Department of Radiation Oncology, Brigham and Women's Hospital and Dana Farber Cancer Institute, Boston, MA.
Morote J	jmorote@vhebron.net	Translational Prostate Cancer Research Program, Vall d'Hebron Hospital, Autónoma University, Medical School, Barcelona, Spain
Moul JW	jmoul@cpdr.org	Department of Surgery, Center for Prostate Disease Research, Uniformed Services University of the Health Sciences, Bethesda, Maryland 20852, US
Mucci LA	lmucci@hsph.harvard.edu	Channing Laboratory, Brigham and Women's Hospital and Harvard Medical School, Boston, MA 02115,
Naito S	naito@uresino.hosp.go.jp	Division of Pathology, Research Laboratory, National Hospital Organization, Ureshino Medical Center, Saga, Japan
Nakagawa K	nakagawa@igm.hokudai.ac.jp	Division of Cancer Gene Regulation, Research Section of Disease Control, Institute for Genetic Medicine, Hokkaido University, Sapporo 060-0815, Japan
Namiki S	namikin@uro.med.tohoku.ac.jp	Department of Urology, Tohoku University Graduate School of Medicine, Sendai, Japan,
Neal DE	den22@cam.ac.uk	Department of Oncology, University of Cambridge, Cambridge CB2 0QQ, UK

Name	Email	Institution
Nelson C	nelsonc@mskcc.org	Memorial Sloan-Kettering Cancer Center, New York, NY, USA
Nelson PS	psnels@u.washington.edu	Department of Urology, University of Washington, Seattle, WA 98195, USA.
Nelson WG	bnelson@jhmi.edu	Sidney Kimmel Comprehensive Cancer Center, Johns Hopkins University School of Medicine, Baltimore, Maryland 21231-1000, USA
Neuhouser ML	mneuhous@fhcrc.org	Cancer Prevention Program, Division of Public Health Sciences, Fred Hutchinson Cancer Research Center, Seattle, WA 98109-1024, USA.r
Nguyen PL	pnguyen@LROC.harvard.edu	Harvard Radiation Oncology Program, Boston, MA 02115, USA
Nogueira L	nogueirl@mskcc.org	Department of Surgery, Memorial Sloan-Kettering Cancer Center, New York, NY 10065 , USA
Oh WK	william_oh@dfci.harvard.edu	Dana-Farber Cancer Institute, Harvard Medical School, Boston, MA.
Pienta KJ	kpienta@umich.edu	Department of Internal Medicine, University of Michigan Comprehensive Cancer Center, Ann Arbor, Michigan 48109, USA
Piroth MD	marc.piroth@rwth-aachen.de	Department of Radiation Oncology, RWTH Aachen University, Aachen, Germany.
Pisters LL	Lpisters@mdanderson.org	Department of Pathology, The University of Texas M D Anderson Cancer Center, Houston, TX 77030-4009, USA.
Platz EA	eplatz@jhsph.edu	Department of Epidemiology, Johns Hopkins Bloomberg School of Public Health, the James Buchanan Brady Urological Institute, and the Sidney Kimmel Comprehensive Cancer Center, Johns Hopkins Medical Institutions, Baltimore, Maryland 21205
Ploussard G	g.ploussard@gmail.com	INSERM U955 EQ07, Departments of Urology and Pathology, APHP, CHU Henri Mondor, Créteil, France.
Polascik TJ	polas001@mc.duke.edu	Division of Urology, Department of Surgery, Duke University Medical Center, Durham, NC
Pollack A	A_Pollack@FCCC.edu	Department of Radiation Oncology, Fox Chase Cancer Center, 333 Cottman Ave, Philadelphia, PA 19111-2497, USA
Roobol MJ	m.roobol@erasmusmc.nl	Department of Urology, Erasmus Medical Center, Rotterdam, The Netherlands, www.eur.nl/english/
Rosser CJ	charles.rosser@urology.ufl.edu	Department of Urology and Pharmacology and Therapeutics, University of Florida, Gainesville, Florida, USA
Roupret M	mroupret@club-internet.fr	Service d'Urologie Hôpital Pitié-Salpétrière, AP-HP, Groupe Hospitalo-Universitaire Est, 47-83 boulevard de l'Hôpital, 75651 Paris cedex 13, France.
Rubben H	herbert.ruebben@uni-essen.de	Urologische Klinik und Poliklinik, Universitätsklinikum Essen, Essen, Deutschland.
Schalken JA	j.schalken@uro.umcn.nl	Department of Urology, 267 Experimental Urology, Radboud University Nijmegen Medical Centre, PO Box 9101, NL-6500HB Nijmegen, The Netherlands
Schroder FH	e.vandenberg@erasmusmc.nl	Department of Urology, Erasmus Medical Center, Rotterdam, The Netherlands, www.eur.nl/english/

List 1. Alphabetical list of top ranked participants for year 2009 (page 6)

Name	Email	Institution
Severi G	gianluca.severi@cancervic.org.au	Cancer Epidemiology Centre, The Cancer Council Victoria, Carlton, Victoria 3053, Australia.
Shah RB	rajshah@umich.edu	Department of Pathology, University of Michigan, Ann Arbor, MI 48109, USA
Stark JR	stark@hsph.harvard.edu	Department of Epidemiology, Harvard School of Public Health, 677 Huntington Avenue, Boston, MA 02115, USA
Stattin P	par.stattin@urologi.umu.se	Department of Surgical and Perioperative Sciences, Urology and Andrology, Umeå University, Umeå, Sweden.
Stenman UH	ulf-hakan.stenman@helsinki.fi	Department of Clinical Chemistry, Biomedicum Helsinki, University of Helsinki, Helsinki University Central Hospital, Helsinki, Finland.
Stephan C	carsten.stephan@charite.de	Department of Urology, Charite-Universitätsmedizin Berlin, Berlin, Germany.
Stephenson AJ	stephea2@ccf.org	Glickman Urological and Kidney Institute, Cleveland Clinic, Cleveland, Ohio, USA
Sternberg CN	cstern@mclink.it	Department of Medical Oncology, San Camillo and Forlanini Hospitals, Nuovi Padiglioni, 4th Floor, Circonvallazione Gianicolense 87, IT-00152, Rome, Italy
Steuber T	steuber@uke.uni-hamburg.de	Department of Urology, University Clinic Hamburg Eppendorf, Hamburg, Germany
Steyerberg EW	e.steyerberg@erasmusmc.nl	Department of Urology, Erasmus Medical Center, Rotterdam, The Netherlands, www.eur.nl/english/
Stone NN	nelsonstone@optonline.net	Mount Sinai School of Medicine, New York, NY, USA
Tamura K	hiro@ps.toyaku.ac.jp	Department of Endocrine Pharmacology, Tokyo University of Pharmacy & Life Sciences, Horinouchi 1432-1, Hachioji, Tokyo, 192-0392, Japan
Thompson IM	thompsoni@uthscsa.edu	Division of Urology, Beth Israel Deaconess Medical Center, Boston, Massachusetts 20015
Tomlins SA	tomlinss@med.umich.edu	Department of Pathology, University of Michigan Medical School, Ann Arbor, Michigan 48109, USA
van den Bergh RC	r.vandenbergh@erasmusmc.nl	Department of Urology, Erasmus MC, University Medical Center, Rotterdam, The Netherlands.
van der Kwast TH	theo.vdkwast@uhn.on.ca	Department of Pathology and Laboratory Medicine, Mount Sinai Hospital and University Health Network, Toronto, Canada.
Van Der Poel HG	h.vd.poel@nki.nl	Department of Urology, Netherlands Cancer Institute, Plesmanlaan 121, 1066 CX Amsterdam, The Netherlands
van Leenders GJ	G.vanleenders@pathol.azn.nl	Department of Urology, Erasmus Medical Center, Rotterdam, The Netherlands, www.eur.nl/english/
van Vulpen M	M.vanVulpen@UMCUtrecht.nl	Department of Radiation-Oncology, University Medical Center Utrecht, Utrecht, The Netherlands.
Vickers AJ	vickersa@mskcc.org	Department of Epidemiology and Biostatistics, Memorial Sloan-Kettering Cancer Center, New York, New York 10021

List 1. Alphabetical list of top ranked participants for year 2009 (page 7)

Name	Email	Institution
Villers A	a-villers@chru-lille.fr	Urologie, Hôpital Huriez, CHRU 59037 Lille Cedex
Virtamo J	jarmo.virtamo@ktl.fi	National Public Health Institute, Helsinki, Finland
Wiklund F	fredrik.wiklund@oc.umu.se	Department of Radiation Sciences, Oncology, University of Umeå, Umeå, Sweden.
Witjes JA	f.witjes@uro.umcn.nl	Department of Urology, Radboud University Nijmegen Medical Centre, PO Box 9101, 6500 HB Nijmegen, The Netherlands.

Table 1. Country rank for year 2009/ top 124 researchers (List 1), identified by repetitive e-mail counts in PubMed (2,000 set, Appendix A).

Country	Address hits
USA	26
Netherlands	12
Germany	12
Italy	8
Sweden	8
UK	6
Helsinki	5
France	5
Australia	4
Canada	3
Israel	2
Singapore	2

124 addresses analyzed (www.wordle.net), see the 'word-cloud' next page >

Word-cloud for year 2009 top 124 researchers (List 1)

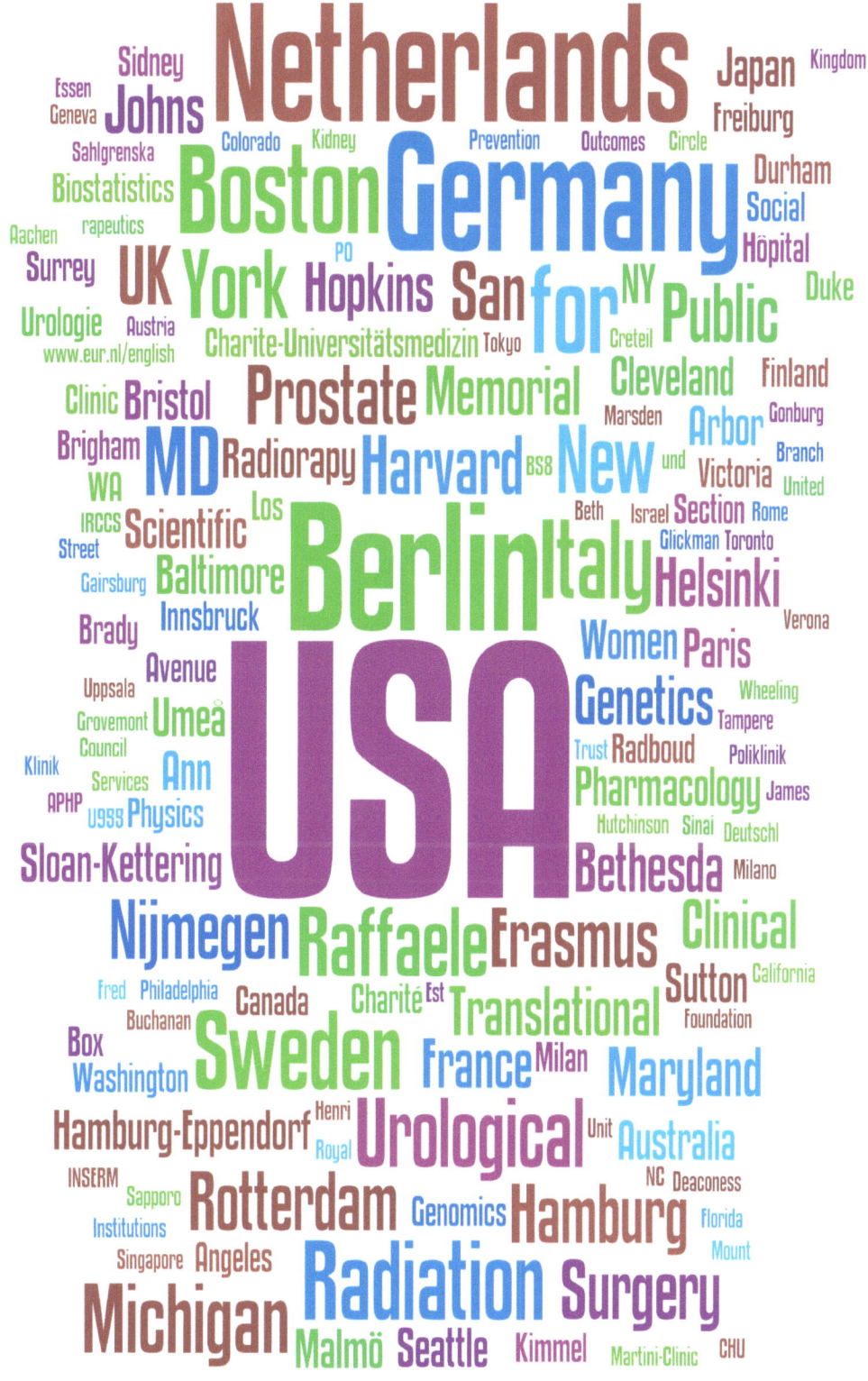

19960500	19937597	19914774	19895682	19866469	19843684	19821979
19960430	19937596	19914773	19895521	19866465	19843661	19821209
19959826	19937163	19914772	19895183	19866464	19843189	19820934
19959505	19937135	19914771	19894759	19864529	19842040	19820397
19959380	19937055	19914769	19893516	19864083	19841937	19820037
19959199	19936421	19914697	19893261	19864082	19841280	19819854
19959000	19936334	19914662	19893039	19864076	19841273	19819536
19957321	19935797	19914651	19892841	19864003	19841101	19819277
19956956	19935788	19914392	19892808	19864001	19840510	19819096
19956877	19935771	19914133	19892375	19863859	19840198	19818764
19956859	19935718	19914107	19891778	19863851	19839735	19818734
19956850	19935713	19914098	19891595	19863624	19839428	19818082
19956848	19935671	19914096	19891594	19863532	19839427	19818078
19956834	19935058	19913885	19890632	19863531	19839426	19818074
19956729	19934913	19913824	19890158	19863529	19839425	19817979
19956567	19934397	19913814	19890017	19863528	19839424	19817747
19956271	19934328	19913499	19889975	19863524	19838855	19817744
19956194	19934327	19913350	19889581	19863523	19838837	19816779
19956193	19934320	19913257	19889223	19863522	19838218	19816598
19955594	19934305	19913252	19889066	19863521	19838216	19816388
19955592	19933651	19913249	19889065	19863420	19838145	19816162
19955085	19933153	19913246	19888981	19863346	19838047	19816159
19954971	19933109	19913184	19888980	19863187	19837689	19815968
19954892	19933031	19913001	19888979	19861995	19837667	19815745
19954284	19932151	19912640	19888978	19861965	19837617	19815622
19953931	19931979	19912486	19888973	19861539	19837616	19815488
19953666	19931977	19912212	19888970	19861534	19837615	19815487
19952762	19931928	19912210	19888874	19861522	19837614	19815486
19952760	19931898	19912205	19888723	19861519	19837527	19815485
19952715	19931892	19912202	19888630	19861517	19837467	19815482
19951953	19931639	19912186	19888222	19861512	19837418	19815259
19951614	19931126	19912185	19888221	19860936	19837417	19815255
19951446	19930869	19912180	19888195	19860934	19837201	19815066
19951257	19930682	19912179	19887948	19860933	19837161	19814782
19950222	19930650	19912094	19887945	19860930	19836968	19814618
19950034	19930334	19911260	19887874	19860842	19836876	19813273
19949849	19930177	19911247	19887614	19860409	19836809	19812222
19949676	19930176	19910554	19887604	19858401	19836806	19811950
19949428	19930175	19910504	19887582	19858385	19836804	19811770
19949374	19930174	19910433	19887552	19858377	19836800	19811656
19949260	19928101	19910427	19887483	19857789	19836788	19811645
19949016	19928099	19910135	19886863	19857260	19836787	19811549
19948822	19926949	19909795	19886716	19857185	19836778	19811499
19948436	19926948	19909775	19885928	19857055	19836774	19811095
19948393	19926941	19908944	19885853	19856978	19836772	19810492
19948241	19926709	19908238	19885850	19856921	19836767	19810487
19948237	19926708	19908237	19885807	19856314	19836757	19810472
19948028	19926313	19908230	19885645	19856060	19836166	19810465
19947927	19926312	19906923	19885619	19855844	19836164	19810463
19947826	19926311	19906782	19885603	19855435	19836161	19810103

Appendix A (page 2, 351-700)

19947776	19925815	19906484	19885599	19855158	19836155	19809978
19947572	19925755	19906297	19885585	19855155	19836060	19809561
19947569	19925754	19904616	19885571	19855091	19835862	19809428
19947562	19925616	19904497	19885564	19854604	19835577	19808972
19947349	19925394	19904272	19885309	19854524	19834822	19808968
19947348	19925393	19904264	19884533	19854485	19834284	19808637
19947347	19925392	19903903	19884383	19854484	19833726	19807203
19946787	19924796	19903888	19884290	19854477	19832994	19806852
19946707	19924305	19903769	19884078	19854473	19832925	19806595
19946604	19924093	19903767	19884031	19854148	19832923	19806465
19946339	19923922	19903718	19883806	19853957	19832922	19806413
19946220	19922545	19903468	19883429	19853940	19832899	19806380
19945997	19922544	19903362	19883296	19853534	19832893	19806320
19945666	19921964	19903116	19882799	19853533	19832890	19806171
19945664	19921834	19903091	19882361	19853532	19832888	19806170
19945663	19921446	19903068	19882268	19853487	19831728	19805692
19945310	19921294	19902477	19882157	19853371	19831159	19805682
19945309	19921205	19902474	19882130	19853370	19830810	19805354
19945303	19921202	19902473	19882057	19852272	19830784	19805306
19944755	19920919	19902470	19881959	19852006	19830782	19805305
19944519	19920916	19902467	19881957	19851870	19830550	19805273
19943972	19920825	19902466	19881949	19850885	19830402	19805192
19943207	19920379	19902465	19881538	19850537	19830081	19805094
19943183	19920378	19902378	19880260	19850536	19829728	19804966
19943145	19920237	19902377	19880259	19850036	19829727	19804961
19943130	19920184	19902366	19879812	19847811	19828205	19804948
19942689	19920136	19902169	19879701	19847385	19827538	19804427
19942459	19920114	19901962	19879700	19847141	19827050	19804426
19942268	19920103	19901959	19879698	19846946	19826760	19804424
19942263	19920098	19901958	19879477	19846944	19826362	19802870
19942262	19919713	19901915	19879475	19846929	19826203	19802609
19942188	19919114	19901851	19879470	19846921	19826199	19802499
19942048	19918950	19901020	19879066	19846918	19826053	19802001
19941668	19918800	19900942	19879063	19846905	19826044	19801769
19941262	19918799	19900389	19879061	19846858	19826025	19801219
19940180	19918264	19900376	19878505	19846775	19826019	19801105
19939895	19918263	19900374	19878164	19846468	19825988	19800672
19939760	19918156	19899373	19877619	19846350	19825963	19800578
19939598	19917860	19899258	19876916	19846348	19825885	19800552
19939580	19917571	19899007	19876914	19846139	19825806	19800544
19939578	19917544	19899006	19875340	19845601	19825802	19800142
19939577	19917542	19899005	19875227	19845529	19824968	19800102
19938335	19917478	19898818	19874819	19844660	19824152	19799647
19938042	19917249	19897336	19874631	19844236	19824150	19798124
19938041	19917083	19897268	19874422	19844233	19824149	19798123
19938016	19916735	19897022	19874262	19844197	19824127	19797969
19938014	19915794	19896265	19873936	19843904	19823874	19797414
19938013	19915614	19895737	19866475	19843864	19823725	19797393
19937954	19915386	19895734	19866473	19843851	19822882	19797051
19937735	19914946	19895686	19866472	19843724	19821991	19796750

Appendix A (page 3, 701-1050)

19796718	19773744	19752886	19725823	19700816	19676083	19653726
19796463	19773450	19752089	19725821	19700748	19676082	19653278
19796462	19773449	19751506	19725582	19700655	19676081	19653110
19796456	19773444	19751390	19725410	19700235	19676054	19653109
19796455	19773438	19751264	19725275	19700213	19676045	19652929
19796129	19773269	19751263	19725049	19699645	19675593	19652721
19796063	19773209	19751256	19725034	19699452	19675320	19652704
19796018	19773114	19748692	19725029	19698163	19674994	19652665
19796017	19773112	19748315	19724911	19698051	19674936	19652581
19795463	19773038	19748146	19724904	19697337	19674469	19652292
19795453	19773035	19748143	19724689	19697155	19674167	19652073
19795418	19772879	19747763	19723920	19695936	19673655	19652037
19795373	19772568	19747564	19723918	19695927	19673008	19652036
19795350	19771394	19747478	19722776	19695815	19672905	19652013
19795124	19770843	19747358	19722471	19695789	19672857	19651516
19794990	19770205	19747357	19722212	19695694	19672450	19650748
19794963	19769656	19746787	19721258	19695446	19672449	19650632
19794244	19769655	19746784	19720970	19695439	19672448	19649987
19792969	19768662	19746436	19720969	19694528	19672434	19649507
19792968	19767773	19745696	19720918	19693937	19672431	19649504
19792961	19767761	19744800	19720912	19693651	19671968	19649210
19792959	19767760	19744341	19720908	19693481	19671871	19648535
19790239	19767755	19744336	19720880	19693098	19671866	19648421
19790238	19767754	19743884	19720450	19692971	19671841	19648420
19790237	19767753	19741638	19720303	19692841	19671799	19647979
19790236	19767752	19741607	19720294	19692759	19671770	19647638
19790235	19767707	19741479	19720291	19692323	19671765	19647634
19790234	19767115	19741211	19719532	19692321	19671688	19647628
19790232	19766667	19740617	19719458	19691856	19671672	19647427
19790231	19766339	19740574	19719457	19691137	19671656	19647299
19790230	19766338	19740429	19719456	19691136	19671219	19647296
19789531	19766336	19740412	19719455	19691135	19671000	19647165
19789370	19766252	19739131	19719454	19691128	19670452	19646631
19789348	19765891	19739130	19719453	19691097	19670261	19646629
19789329	19765846	19739128	19719240	19691092	19670249	19646459
19789311	19765454	19739126	19717752	19690867	19670238	19646431
19789216	19764975	19739124	19717225	19690866	19670229	19646263
19789132	19764041	19738609	19717197	19690725	19670224	19645454
19788872	19763400	19738602	19717042	19690611	19670218	19645029
19787785	19763272	19738124	19716895	19690552	19669670	19645025
19787772	19763266	19738114	19716781	19690549	19669099	19644960
19787702	19762612	19738095	19716766	19690545	19668381	19644955
19787636	19762548	19738074	19716591	19690542	19668226	19644954
19787436	19762255	19738069	19716590	19690330	19667269	19644707
19787273	19762048	19738062	19716227	19690196	19667155	19644150
19787268	19762047	19738059	19716160	19690195	19667147	19643837
19787211	19761424	19738047	19715609	19690187	19667145	19643650
19787193	19760800	19738045	19715115	19690186	19667069	19643479
19787003	19760638	19738000	19715036	19690108	19666938	19643467
19786982	19760636	19737984	19714536	19690043	19666904	19643431

Appendix A (page 4, 1051-1400)

19786981	19760632	19737977	19714336	19690023	19666892	19643236
19786681	19760631	19737975	19713972	19689825	19666408	19642913
19786680	19760629	19737972	19713548	19689476	19665390	19642689
19786673	19760628	19737960	19711917	19688826	19665338	19642159
19786659	19760627	19737788	19711916	19686648	19665322	19642108
19785943	19760626	19737411	19711464	19686421	19665286	19641239
19785775	19760433	19737398	19711215	19686355	19665215	19641224
19784964	19760427	19737278	19710042	19686273	19664875	19640766
19784785	19760170	19736919	19709958	19685532	19664817	19640762
19784071	19760149	19736590	19709167	19685053	19664336	19640758
19784068	19759906	19736306	19709074	19684615	19664332	19640722
19783927	19759384	19736046	19709072	19684515	19664134	19640296
19783900	19759109	19735890	19708928	19684076	19664128	19640273
19783378	19759108	19735884	19708043	19683860	19664112	19639606
19783375	19758747	19735867	19707953	19683858	19664042	19639466
19782069	19758683	19735466	19707524	19683763	19663894	19639414
19782051	19758657	19735258	19707199	19683746	19663810	19639194
19781848	19758646	19735167	19707172	19683745	19663790	19639176
19781751	19758645	19734935	19706948	19683743	19663730	19639174
19781746	19758638	19734774	19706860	19683737	19663697	19639170
19781717	19758635	19734683	19706848	19683667	19662653	19638584
19781100	19758625	19734106	19706844	19683515	19662405	19638540
19780165	19758620	19734069	19706826	19683331	19661793	19638505
19780158	19758618	19734068	19706820	19683310	19661570	19638463
19779961	19758616	19734067	19706804	19683305	19661347	19638459
19779262	19758611	19733987	19706803	19683299	19661342	19638458
19779119	19758610	19733959	19706801	19683287	19661323	19638457
19779093	19757659	19733126	19706800	19683286	19661078	19638245
19779034	19757658	19733014	19706777	19683274	19661028	19638170
19778971	19757530	19733013	19706771	19683269	19660851	19637935
19778970	19757253	19732746	19706764	19683262	19660791	19637357
19778969	19756851	19732303	19706750	19683261	19659898	19637345
19778537	19756633	19732065	19706031	19682889	19659608	19637339
19778521	19756592	19732053	19705986	19682790	19659465	19637245
19778174	19756426	19731262	19705979	19681902	19657768	19637042
19777538	19756425	19731191	19705489	19681901	19657379	19636411
19777359	19755998	19731129	19705098	19681898	19657377	19636237
19777185	19755987	19730863	19704984	19681044	19657376	19636023
19776696	19755982	19730362	19704337	19680997	19657374	19636017
19776002	19755981	19730351	19703998	19680621	19657348	19635998
19775849	19755699	19728195	19703883	19680620	19657239	19635783
19775826	19755655	19728173	19703854	19680443	19657228	19635642
19775807	19755651	19728119	19703789	19679405	19655267	19634174
19775659	19755645	19727818	19703300	19679054	19654868	19634073
19775638	19754693	19727241	19701842	19678840	19654575	19634072
19775632	19754215	19727148	19701634	19678815	19654307	19633975
19775615	19754211	19727147	19701499	19678799	19654297	19633685
19775613	19754210	19727146	19701241	19676109	19654133	19633053
19775154	19754130	19727145	19701218	19676095	19653896	19633050
19773757	19753950	19726753	19701187	19676093	19653874	19633045

Appendix A (page 5, 1401-1700)

19632246	19597029	19562346	19507253	19437533	19338564
19632176	19596255	19560453	19507229	19437096	19338553
19632069	19594895	19560260	19507201	19436213	19338545
19632009	19594741	19560140	19506163	19434660	19332512
19629986	19594734	19559785	19506162	19434657	19330328
19629981	19594731	19559507	19506151	19434652	19326171
19629969	19594367	19559437	19506150	19434633	19326061
19628766	19593854	19558577	19505431	19433685	19322680
19628521	19593853	19558559	19503095	19433345	19320614
19628502	19593852	19556867	19503093	19433338	19319526
19628258	19593851	19556345	19501880	19433067	19308411
19627283	19593850	19556286	19501628	19433066	19303721
19627282	19593773	19556072	19501454	19431146	19301006
19626664	19593445	19555350	19499262	19430785	19298408
19626653	19592505	19554630	19497389	19430782	19298406
19626590	19592154	19554503	19496069	19430494	19297146
19625770	19592122	19553822	19496068	19428311	19289266
19625447	19592075	19553817	19496055	19428310	19289254
19625182	19591615	19553641	19495832	19428309	19286370
19625136	19591186	19552894	19495772	19428071	19285710
19625135	19591135	19551858	19495750	19428067	19282812
19625061	19590529	19549509	19494112	19428064	19282170
19624852	19589791	19549261	19493624	19428062	19281468
19624845	19589639	19549256	19493248	19427875	19281464
19624597	19589584	19549252	19492418	19427750	19281463
19624596	19589580	19547971	19492334	19427017	19280188
19624594	19589573	19546404	19491931	19426197	19278776
19624592	19589569	19545787	19489038	19426190	19277882
19624535	19589564	19545597	19489030	19426187	19277881
19624098	19589167	19544444	19489029	19424758	19272866
19623543	19588525	19544409	19489028	19423179	19269808
19623542	19588362	19544327	19488063	19422047	19269165
19622840	19588206	19543955	19487148	19422046	19268572
19622774	19588120	19543735	19487081	19421755	19267250
19622756	19587348	19541487	19487074	19418497	19263441
19622584	19586654	19541477	19486654	19418243	19263243
19622577	19585579	19541463	19484790	19415749	19254280
19621387	19585577	19540305	19484788	19415730	19250768
19620493	19585501	19540077	19483730	19415690	19250761
19620481	19585491	19539327	19483721	19415464	19247669
19619961	19585490	19538337	19482075	19414670	19246230
19619960	19585401	19536890	19481922	19410316	19245439
19619065	19584328	19536889	19481336	19409691	19243900
19619056	19584279	19536794	19479898	19409690	19242732
19619001	19584168	19536097	19479278	19409636	19239458
19618377	19584163	19535981	19479252	19409635	19239451
19618291	19584087	19535293	19477898	19408303	19239447
19617846	19584056	19535108	19477747	19407851	19239443
19616957	19583812	19535105	19477736	19406609	19234708
19616901	19583731	19535005	19477172	19406240	19233568

Appendix A (page 6, 1701-2000)

19616835	19583720	19533748	19476985	19406209	19225888
19616830	19583717	19533723	19476981	19403241	19221747
19616799	19582846	19533582	19476978	19402094	19220271
19616746	19582786	19530253	19475654	19399788	19220264
19616743	19582779	19530242	19475643	19399787	19220263
19616286	19581923	19530240	19475640	19399749	19220260
19616281	19581582	19530225	19475570	19399647	19220251
19616279	19581310	19529978	19474291	19398902	19217022
19616262	19580824	19528873	19474090	19398328	19214529
19616259	19579185	19528667	19473376	19396604	19214504
19616258	19579052	19528666	19470933	19395198	19214393
19616228	19578936	19528373	19470632	19395194	19212706
19616226	19578797	19528369	19470463	19395188	19211196
19616162	19578775	19526991	19468736	19395184	19205910
19616157	19578773	19524984	19467856	19394814	19201267
19615834	19578772	19524966	19467803	19393705	19201081
19615826	19578741	19524963	19467571	19393638	19197947
19615720	19578724	19524953	19466946	19389811	19185987
19615679	19578386	19524545	19466945	19389009	19184473
19610065	19578160	19524478	19466429	19389007	19180530
19610059	19578133	19524036	19465015	19388988	19172579
19609570	19578042	19523704	19464826	19388987	19167919
19609297	19577865	19522869	19464820	19388986	19167839
19608952	19577864	19522868	19464745	19387639	19156675
19608864	19577859	19522739	19463689	19386460	19147306
19608857	19577562	19522464	19462989	19386427	19142636
19608787	19577536	19522014	19462463	19384952	19137527
19608712	19576799	19521962	19460858	19380442	19131185
19608628	19576798	19521959	19459176	19377857	19131179
19608618	19576796	19520982	19459159	19376571	19117691
19607725	19576760	19520795	19457625	19376570	19115108
19606178	19575788	19520778	19457353	19375907	19104815
19605506	19575420	19520769	19455605	19375853	19084352
19603378	19574450	19519765	19454624	19375825	19058919
19603032	19574343	19517575	19453917	19375269	19051034
19603015	19574101	19517474	19452568	19375243	19022265
19602280	19573808	19517223	19450551	19375217	19005751
19602258	19573625	19517139	19448671	19373471	18931824
19602007	19572116	19515843	19447103	19373278	18926679
19602006	19571228	19515794	19446546	19370395	18848788
19602005	19569252	19515504	19445482	19363437	18824345
19602004	19568772	19515403	19444909	19362783	18773296
19601677	19568244	19515209	19444856	19362044	18718111
19598210	19565568	19515173	19444819	19358991	18639471
19597915	19564094	19514049	19444304	19357389	18625570
19597533	19562736	19513720	19444125	19352653	18625566
19597474	19562734	19513599	19443907	19345517	18625565
19597471	19562729	19513068	19442516	19345515	18583166
19597470	19562724	19512934	19439180	19342698	18534873
19597465	19562712	19509068	19438509	19340595	18516691